HYPERTENSION TREATMENT: USER GUIDE

Second Edition

by

Norman M. Kaplan, M.D.

Department of Internal Medicine
University of Texas
Southwestern Medical School
5323 Harry Hines Boulevard
Dallas, Texas 75235

Essential Medical

Information Systems, Inc.

P.O. Box 1607

Durant, Oklahoma 74702

For orders, please call:
1-800-225-0694

Published in the United States 1993

ISBN: 0-929240-53-7

Second Edition

36108

Printed in the United States of America

New and Updated Center Index Texts
Published By
Essential Medical Information Systems, Inc.

A Practical Anesthesia Information Guide —*Jerome*

Emergency Cardiac Maneuvers — 2nd Ed. —*Bartecchi*

Management of Hypertension — 4th Ed. —*Kaplan*

Contraceptive Surgery For Men and Women — 2nd Ed. — *Moss/AVSC*

Managing Contraceptive Pill Patients — 6th Ed. —*Dickey*

Breastfeeding: *A Problem-Solving Manual* —3rd Ed. — *Saunders, Carroll & Johnson*

Management of Infertility: *A Clinician's Manual* —2nd Ed. — *Cohen*

Cholesterol Treatment: *User Guide To Lipid Disorder Management* —2nd Ed. —*Leaf*

Arthritis Therapy: *A Clinician's Manual* —*Kantor*

Management of Heart Failure —*Cohn & Kubo*

Menopause: *Clinical Concepts* —*London & Chihal*

Premenstrual Syndrome —2nd Ed. —*Chihal*

Management of Diabetes Mellitus —2nd Ed. —*Schwartz*

Managing Danazol Patients —2nd Ed. —*Dickey*

Hormone Replacement Therapy —3rd Ed. —*Gambrell*

Endometriosis: *The Enigmatic Disease* —*Corson*

Mid Life Sexuality: *Enrichment & Problem Solving* —*Semmens*

A Manual on Drug Dependence — *Nahas*

Projective Psychodiagnostic Assessment —*Caldwell & Dixon*

TABLE OF CONTENTS

What is Hypertension?
The Normal Blood Pressure 8
What do the Numbers Mean? 12
Why Does the Blood Pressure Go Up? 16
What are the Consequences of
     High Blood Pressure? 24
Can Hypertension Be Prevented? 28

Treating Hypertension Without Drugs
Overview of Non-Drug Treatment 30
Weight Reduction 34
Moderate Sodium Restriction 40
Extra Potassium, Calcium, Magnesium 44
Fiber and Fats, Alcohol and Caffeine 48
Exercise 50
Relaxation 52

Treating Hypertension With Drugs
General Guidelines 54
An Overview of Drug Treatment 56
Diuretics and Potassium Sparers 64
Sympathetic Blockers: Peripheral
     and Central 70
Sympathetic Blockers: Alpha and Beta 74
Calcium Entry Blockers 76
Angiotensin Converting Enzyme
     (ACE) Inhibitors 78
Other Antihypertensive Drugs 80

Treating Special People and Problems
Diabetics 82
Heart Disease 84
Cerebral Disease 86
Kidney Disease 88
Impotence and Other Symptoms 90
Elderly 92
Children 94

Taking Your Own Blood Pressure 96

TABLES

TABLE 3.1 — Sodium Content of
Common Foods 21
TABLE 3.2 — Causes and Tests for
Secondary Hypertension 23
TABLE 6.1 — Overall Non-Drug Program 33
TABLE 7.1 — How to Figure Your
"Ideal Weight" 38
TABLE 7.2 — Example of Reasonable
Weight-Loss Program 39
TABLE 8.1 — Sodium Content of Some
Typical Processed Foods 42
TABLE 8.2 — Examples of Low-Sodium
Substitutes for High-Sodium Foods 43
TABLE 9.1 — Estimated Diet of Late Paleolithic
Man vs. That of Contemporary Americans   46
TABLE 9.2 — Low-Sodium Foods 47
TABLE 14.1 — Types of Drugs Used to
Treat Hypertension 58
TABLE 15.1 — Diuretics 68
TABLE 16.1 — Characteristics of
Sympathetic Blocker 72

FIGURES

FIGURE 1.1 — Blood Pressures in
Various Parts of the Circulation 10
FIGURE 2.1 — Dial Sphygmomanometer
and Mercury Sphygmomanometer 15
FIGURE 4.1 — The Natural History of
Untreated Essential Hypertension 26
FIGURE 4.2 — The Danger of Heart
Attack and Stroke 27
FIGURE 11.1 — The Effects of Isometric
Exercise in a Hypertensive Person 51
FIGURE 14.1 — The Effects of
Antihypertensive Medications on
the Blood Pressure 60
FIGURE 26.1 — Prevalence of Hypertension
With Advancing Age 93

The Treatment of High Blood Pressure

Foreword

Over 40 million Americans have high blood pressure or hypertension. If you or someone you care about are one of them, this book is designed to provide information to help control this common condition. It should be used along with the advice of your doctor.

This book is written with these goals:

- Replace fear and misinformation which can aggravate your blood pressure problem with facts that should help relieve stress, which is one of the causes for an elevated pressure
- Provide guidance for the individual who wants to lower blood pressure without drugs through diet, exercise, relaxation and other proven methods
- Give the information needed to help your doctor treat you effectively with antihypertensive medications. In particular, common side effects such as weakness, easy fatigue and impotence will be addressed so they may be avoided

As a better informed patient, you can be an effective partner with your physician in changing what used to be "the silent killer" into an easily managed condition.

#1 The Normal Blood Pressure

The circulation can be looked upon as a pump (heart) and a series of tubes (arteries, capillaries and veins) filled with fluid (blood) (Figure 1.1).

Compare the circulation to your outdoor lawn sprinkler system: the pump is a large one owned by the city but you have a spigot which you can open to varying degrees to let water enter your system, the spigot acting like the heart. You attach a fairly thick hose to the spigot serving as an artery to lead water to the sprinkler heads which provide small drips of water where it is needed, just as the tiny capillaries bring blood with oxygen, glucose and other needed nutrients to the various organs of the body. Since the body recycles the same fluid constantly, there are tubes (veins) collecting the blood from the organs, returning it to the heart so it can be pumped out again after being revitalized by going through the lungs where waste products are removed and oxygen added.

The pressure in your sprinkler system depends upon the:

- Amount of pressure generated by the city pump (the force of the heart beat)
- Degree that the spigot is opened (the frequency of the heart beat)
- Size of the garden hose (the diameter of the arteries)
- Settings in the sprinkler heads (the diameter of the capillaries)

Obviously, pressure can be too high which can cause the pipes to burst or too low which prevents water from getting to your lawn. As we shall see, the same principles apply to the human circulation. Ordinarily you do not worry about the pressure in your sprinkler system, as long as there are no leaks or other problems. However, we cannot wait for problems to occur in our circulatory system, so we do measure the pressure.

The place where the pressure within the circulation is most easily measured in the human body is over the large artery (the brachial artery) in the upper arm just above or below the elbow. Since it is close to the heart, the pressure in the brachial artery is similar to what is in the heart and major artery (the aorta) that leads from it. The pressure falls considerably as the arteries break up into capillaries within the organs and there is just enough pressure left in the veins to get the blood back to the heart.

Your blood pressure, then, is related to the strength and rate of your heart (cardiac output) and the size or tightness of your arteries (peripheral resistance).

FIGURE 1.1 BLOOD PRESSURES IN VARIOUS PARTS OF THE CIRCULATION

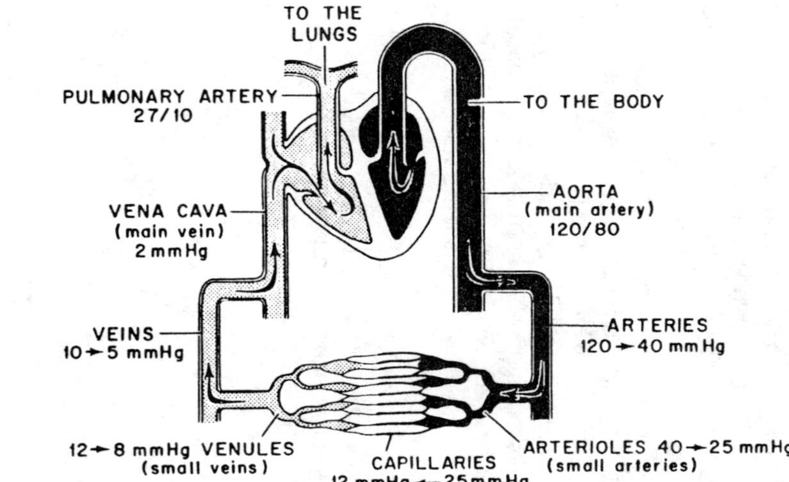

FIGURE 1.1—A schematized view of the heart and blood vessels showing the levels of pressure in various parts of the circulation.

NOTES

#2 What Do the Numbers Mean?

Your heart is an exceedingly efficient pump, activated by a self-generated electrical impulse. With each beat, a little more than two ounces of blood are squeezed from your heart into your large arteries, and this occurs about 70 times a minute. (That is over 100,000 times a day, which can be multiplied into a fantastic number of heart-beats over a lifetime — about 2.5 billion.) The pressure built up by this sudden outflow of blood from the heart into the large arteries is the higher number of your blood pressure reading, referred to as the systolic pressure. Systole is the medical term for the period of heart contraction. As the blood flows out of the arteries into the tissues, the pressure within the arteries gradually falls. The lowest pressure reached, just before the next heartbeat, is the lower number of your blood pressure reading, the diastolic pressure. Diastole is the medical term for the period of heart relaxation between each heartbeat.

The Measurement of Blood Pressure

The device used to measure the blood pressure is called a sphygmomanometer (Figure 2.1). (Electronic blood pressure measuring devices are now available which you can use to do it much easier, but the principles are the same). This device is comprised of two major parts:
- A balloon encased in a rigid cuff which encircles your arm
- A gauge to measure the pressure within the cuff

Air is pumped into the balloon until the pressure of the balloon on your arm is greater than the pressure within the large artery in your arm. The higher pressure temporarily stops the flow of blood into your arm through the artery, as can be recognized by the disappearance of your pulse. The temporary stoppage of blood flow should cause no discomfort (if the balloon were kept inflated for some minutes, however, your arm would begin to ache).

The person taking your blood pressure puts a sound amplifier (usually a stethoscope) over the region just below the elbow crease where the artery is located. The pressure in the balloon is slowly released by opening a valve. When the pressure in the balloon falls below the upper level of your blood pressure (the systolic pressure), a spurt of blood escapes from the constricted artery below the balloon with each heartbeat. This blood entering your forearm produces a thumping sound in the stethoscope. (The electronic blood-pressure devices use a microphone or oscilloscope to pick up this noise and display the number or beep the sound.) The level of your blood pressure when this thumping sound begins is your systolic blood pressure, which can be read as a result of its effect against either a column of mercury or an air gauge. The pressure is expressed in millimeters of mercury (mm Hg), which would be the height to which your blood pressure would push a column of mercury. The normal systolic pressure is about 120 millimeters of mercury (120 mm Hg).

After the upper level of pressure is noted, more air in the balloon is released so that more blood flows into your forearm, continuing to produce the thumping sound. When the pressure in the balloon falls below the lower level of your blood pressure, there is no further obstruction of blood flow, and the sound in your artery disappears. This level is the diastolic blood pressure and is normally about 80 mm Hg.

The result is a normal blood pressure of about 120 over 80 millimeters of mercury, expressed as 120/80 mm Hg. The normal level is much lower in infancy and childhood, reaching adult levels at the time of physical maturity. Everyone's blood pressure varies from time to time. If your blood pressure is usually high, it may vary even more. Do not be surprised if readings taken just minutes apart are 10 to 20 mm Hg different. Some of these differences may be due to excitement, nervousness, physical activity or even the time of day. During sleep your blood pressure tends to be much lower than when you are awake.

Even an occasional high reading should not be ignored because it may be a warning signal that more persistent hypertension is developing. Fortunately, attention to certain factors (see Section #3) may stop the rise in pressure if hypertension is recognized early.

Taking Your Own Blood Pressure

More and more physicians are asking patients to take their own pressure at home, at work, and particularly at certain times:

- early in the morning, soon after arising. This is the time when most heart attacks and strokes occur and it is important to know that the pressure is not too high at this time
- anytime symptoms of too high or too low pressure are noted
- whenever medication is changed, to ensure that it is working well throughout the entire day

What you need to know about taking your own pressure is described in Section #28.

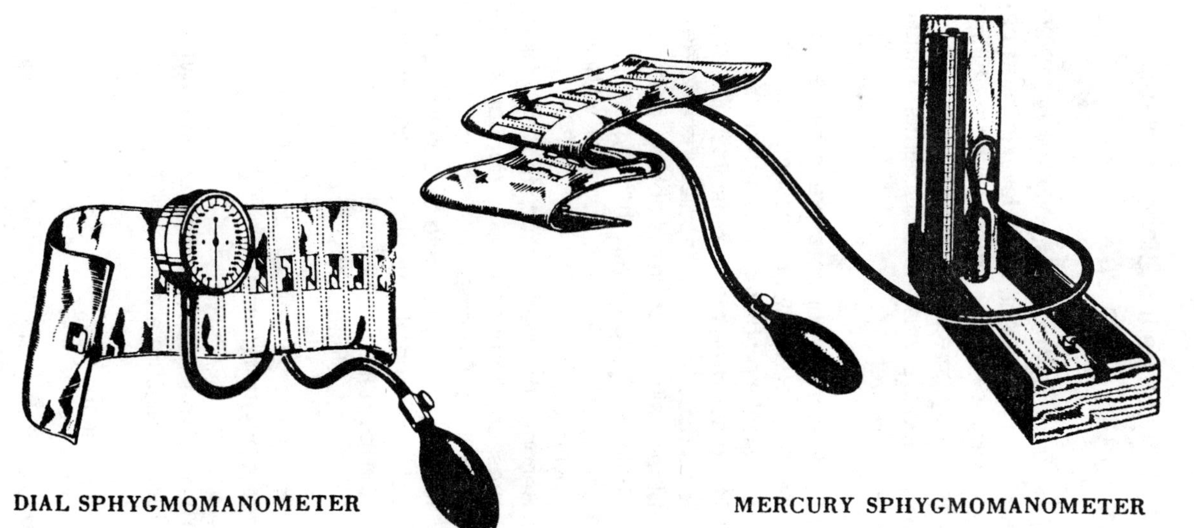

FIGURE 2.1 — (A) Dial sphygmomanometer and (B) mercury sphygmomanometer.

#3 Why Does the Blood Pressure Go Up?

If the readings are persistently above 140/90, hypertension is present. That level is used because the risks of heart and vascular problems are significantly increased if pressures above 140/90 are allowed to persist. Two disclaimers should be noted, however:

- First, even if your pressure is higher than 140/90, you will not necessarily have heart or vascular problems and you may not need immediate treatment. Most vascular problems occur in those people who also have other risks, such as smoking and high cholesterol, along with their hypertension. You should, however, consult with your physician
- Second, the risks associated with blood pressure do not suddenly appear at 140/90. If your normal reading is 110/70, a reading of 130/85 could be a warning signal. In general, the higher your reading above normal, the more likely you need to bring your blood pressure down

Causes of Hypertension

The three names for the most common type of high blood pressure are:

- Essential
- Primary
- Idiopathic

Although the cause is unknown for this type of hypertension, four factors seem to be involved:

- Heredity
- Obesity
- Sodium in the diet
- Psychological stress

We will examine each cause, starting with the only one that cannot be changed — heredity.

Heredity

A tendency or predisposition to develop high blood pressure is passed on from parent to child. The reasons for this are unknown, but we do know that if one or both of your parents had hypertension, your chances of developing high blood pressure are about twice those of a person without a hypertensive parent.

Since we have no way at present of identifying the gene or genes involved, we urge children and other relatives of hypertensive persons to have their blood pressure checked yearly and to be aware of the factors causing high blood pressure mentioned previously that *can* be controlled.

Obesity

Overweight children and adults are twice as likely to have hypertension as people of normal weight. Why obesity causes the pressure to rise is unknown, but we should try to keep children from becoming obese, since there is a strong likelihood that a fat baby will grow into a fat adult. The problem is particularly seen among men who put on "middle-age spread," extra fat in their abdomen and upper body. Unfortunately, this is common in American males and is typically involved in hypertension that begins after age 40.

If you are overweight, loss of weight will probably help reduce your blood pressure. Since this is very important, we will consider it further in Section #7, Weight Reduction.

Sodium in The Diet

Most of us are eating 10 to 20 times the amount of sodium needed. It is likely that this high sodium intake (mostly in the form of table salt, or sodium chloride) is responsible for much of our hypertension.

Salt was first used because it was a good preservative, preventing the growth of food-spoiling bacteria. Before refrigeration was practical, salt curing or pickling were the only ways to preserve meat. Although we now have better ways to preserve foods and the need for salt preservation methods are gone, we have acquired a taste for sodium. Today almost every processed food has sodium added, primarily to make it more palatable. Most canned foods, frozen foods and "fast" foods do not taste salty, but many of them contain large quantities of sodium (Table 3.1).

We are not born with a taste for sodium and we do not need the salt. Breast milk is very low in sodium, but it is obviously adequate for the infant's needs. Yet the average amount of sodium ingested by 1-year-olds in the United States is about five to ten times greater than is necessary. In this way, we develop a life-long preference for sodium. We should reduce this excessive sodium intake, thereby helping to prevent hypertension. Even those who are not hypertensive will probably benefit from a reduction in sodium intake. We will discuss ways to reduce dietary sodium in Section #8, Sodium Restriction.

Psychological Stress

The last of the four factors that may be responsible for your hypertension is a high level of psychological stress. There is less evidence for stress causing hypertension than the other factors. But it has been suggested as one of the reasons why black people, living as a minority and frequently under higher socioeconomic stress, have almost twice as much hypertension as do other persons.

Some people enjoy or even seek stress. But others, perhaps those who "keep it all inside," suffer more heart disease and hypertension. A decreased exposure to stress or better ways of dealing with it may help prevent hypertension and may lower blood pressures that are already too high.

The Role of Alcohol, Tobacco and Cholesterol

In addition to the above-mentioned factors, alcohol may contribute to hypertension. People who drink more than about 1.5 ounces of alcohol a day (as contained in three or more mixed drinks, 4-ounce glasses of wine, or cans of beer) have more hypertension than do those who drink less. However, those who drink no alcohol may have more heart attacks than those who drink in moderation.

Cigarette smoking is bad for your health for many reasons, but it does not seem to cause chronic hypertension. Further, there is no direct relation between high cholesterol or fat intake and hypertension, although those who have an elevated cholesterol level, along with those who smoke cigarettes, are more likely to have early heart disease and strokes. Together with hypertension, high cholesterol intake and cigarette smoking constitute the three largest risk factors for premature cardiovascular disease.

Secondary Hypertension

Your hypertension is probably "essential" or due to unknown causes. About one in 20 cases of hypertension is due to a recognizable cause. These "secondary" forms of hypertension are considered in the evaluation you undergo after your blood pressure has been found to be high. Table 3.2 highlights a few of these secondary causes and the tests used to determine them. Your physician will probably arrange for some screening tests (urine and blood examination) to rule out secondary causes. However, unless there is reason to suspect one of these causes, most additional tests are not necessary. Your doctor must make this decision.

Although there are many other causes of hypertension, they are less common and fairly obvious to a physician. Because a few of them are hereditary, you should tell your physician if you have a relative with a secondary form of hypertension, such as certain types of kidney disease or adrenalin-producing tumors.

TABLE 3.1
SODIUM CONTENT OF COMMON FOODS

FOOD	AMOUNT	SODIUM (mg)	CALORIES (kcal)
Bacon	1 strip	51	30
Cake, commercial			
Angel food	1 piece	66	115
Chocolate frosted	1 piece	131	170
White frosted	1 piece	113	175
Cheese			
American	1 oz	210	119
Camembert, domestic	1 oz	210	89
Cream cheese, natural	1 oz	75	112
Parmesan	1 oz	220	118
Pasteurized processed			
American cheese	1 oz	341	111
Cheese spread	1 oz	488	86
Roquefort	1 oz	210	110
Swiss	1 oz	213	111
Chocolate candy bar, plain	1 bar	33	182
Cold cuts	1 oz	390	91
Cookie, commercial, misc.	1 cookie	60	71
Crab, canned regular	1/4 cup	400	40
Crackers			
Graham	5	94	54
Saltine	5	165	65
Doughnut	1	175	137
Dried beef	1 oz	1290	60
Fish sticks	1 oz	53	52
Frankfurters	1	550	155
French fries, salted	1/2 cup	276	233
Ham	1 oz	330	60
Jell-O	1/2 cup	61	71
Meat, canned	1 oz	370	88
Olives	3	493	50
Pancakes	1 4-inch	191	104
Peanut butter	2 tbsp	182	175
Pickle			
Dill, large	1	714	5
Sweet, chip	1	71	1
Pie, fruit	1/8 of pie	452	385

TABLE 3.1 — (Continued)
SODIUM CONTENT OF COMMON FOODS

FOOD	AMOUNT	SODIUM (mg)	CALORIES (kcal)
Pizza			
Commercial	1 piece	647	245
Homemade	1 piece	729	234
Potato chips	1 oz	102	170
Pot pie			
Beef	1	1024	448
Turkey	1	876	423
Chicken	1	876	510
Pretzels, small	5	252	58
Pudding, commercial			
Chocolate	1/2 cup	155	150
Vanilla	1/2 cup	119	160
Sardines, canned	1 oz	247	61
Sauerkraut	1/2 cup	560	14
Sausage	1 oz	287	104
Soup, canned			
Chicken noodle	1 cup	979	62
Split pea	1 cup	922	142
Vegetable beef	1 cup	1025	77
Spaghetti, canned	1 cup	955	190
Sweet roll	1	195	158
Tomato paste	1/2 cup	50	106
Tuna, regular, in oil	1 oz	240	60
TV dinner			
Beef	1	820	347
Ham	1	1177	307
Pork	1	712	416
Meat loaf	1	1221	366
Swiss steak	1	1075	250
Chicken	1	1083	548
Fish	1	1319	326
Waffle, homemade	1 4-inch section	309	181

(Margie JD, Hunt JC: Living with high blood pressure: the hypertensive diet cookbook, pp. 244-246. Bloomfield, NJ, HLS Press, 1978)

TABLE 3.2 CAUSES AND TESTS FOR SECONDARY HYPERTENSION

CAUSES	TESTS
Damage to kidney function (chronic renal disease)	Blood level of waste products removed by the kidney
Obstruction of blood flow to the kidneys (renovascular hypertension)	Listening for an eddy current (bruit) over the kidneys; X-rays of the kidney by renal scan or arteriogram; Plasma renin assays
Overproduction of hormones made in the adrenal gland: Of cortisol = Cushing's disease Of aldosterone = primary aldosteronism Of adrenalin = pheochromocytoma	Blood and urine levels of these hormones
Obstruction of the major artery (coarctation of the aorta)	Feeling the pulses in the leg; X-rays
Use of estrogen-containing medications (oral contraceptives)	Your history
Use of other drugs: adrenal steroids (cortisol derivatives); adrenalin-like drugs (cold remedies, diet pills); drug abuse (cocaine, PCP, etc.)	Your history

#4 What Are the Consequences Of High Blood Pressure?

The higher your blood pressure is and the longer it remains high, the greater your chance will be of having cardiovascular problems (Figure 4.1). The three major risk factors for both heart attacks and strokes (Figure 4.2) are:

- Hypertension
- Smoking
- High cholesterol

The high pressure acting on the walls of the arteries and veins promotes the development of plaques full of cholesterol and fat in the arteries that lead to these vital organs. In addition, the need to pump blood against such high pressure strains the heart muscle.

Effects on the Brain

The most serious effect is a stroke, or cerebrovascular accident (CVA). A stroke is a sudden loss of function of part of the brain caused by some interference in its blood supply. This may be the result of a blood clot (thrombosis) forming on one of the cholesterol plaques or by the rupture of blood through a weakened artery wall (hemorrhage). In either case, the brain cannot function properly and may cause:

- Sudden weakness
- Paralysis
- Loss of speech
- Loss of other brain functions

Hypertension is a major cause of strokes.

Effects on the Heart

The heart can be damaged when a blood clot cuts off blood supply to part of the heart muscle, causing a heart attack or myocardial infarction (MI). This also occurs more frequently in the blood vessels of the heart (coronary arteries) in which plaques have formed as a result of the repetitive beating of a blood pressure that is too high.

The heart muscle may also suffer from the constant strain of having to pump blood out against the higher level of pressure present in the large arteries. During years of such extra work, the heart muscle enlarges and it may fail, like an overworked pump, if the strain is too great. As a result of heart failure, the heart cannot keep blood moving out into the arteries and beyond, and fluid accumulates behind the heart either in the:

- Lungs, causing breathlessness
- Legs, causing swelling (edema)

Effects on the Kidneys

With long-standing hypertension, the small blood vessels in the kidney may be narrowed progressively so that less blood flows through the kidney. As a result, the kidney tissue suffers and the body wastes normally excreted into the urine begin to build up within the blood. Hypertension is a leading cause of kidney failure.

Other Effects

The blood vessels in other parts of the body may also suffer from the constant high pressure.

Those in the eye are especially susceptible, and thus are often examined for evidence of damage from hypertension. Large blood vessels, such as the aorta, and small blood vessels in the legs are also susceptible to damage from long-standing hypertension.

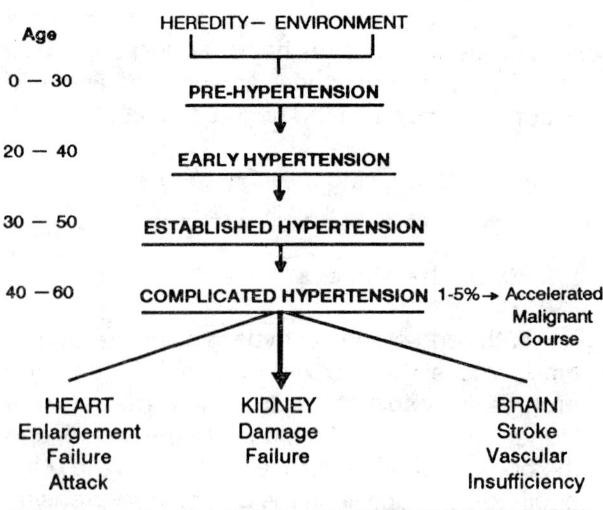

FIGURE 4.1 — The natural history of untreated essential hypertension.

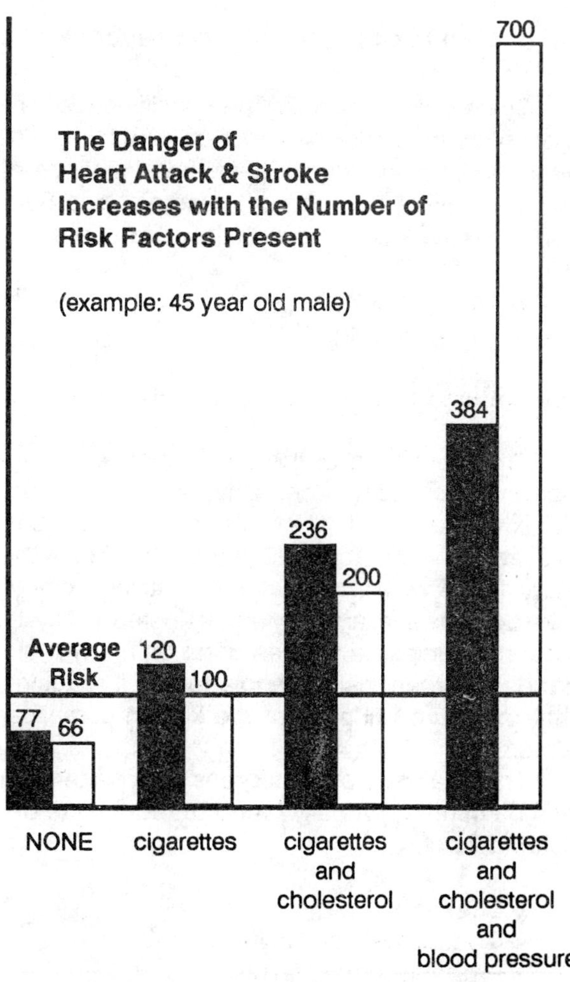

FIGURE 4.2 — The danger of heart attack (solid bar) and stroke (open bar) increases with the number of risk factors present. This diagram shows how a combination of three major risk factors can increase the likelihood of heart attack and stroke. This example uses an abnormal blood pressure level of 180 systolic and a cholesterol level of 310 in a 45-year-old man. (From the Framingham, Massachusetts, Heart Study.)

#5 Can Hypertension Be Prevented?

Since we do not know the specific causes of most hypertension, we cannot be sure hypertension can be prevented. However, avoidance of the three major environmental factors (see Section #3) is a good idea even if they do not prevent hypertension.

We can, however, prevent many of the ill-effects of hypertension.

5. Prevention of Consequences of Hypertension

The prevention of the consequences of hypertension can almost certainly be accomplished. Effective treatment of hypertension has been available only for about 30 years. Starting in the early 1960s when medications relatively easy to take became available (by mouth instead of by injection), studies have been done on many thousands of hypertensive people to see if reducing their pressure will prevent the known complications.

The treatment of all degrees of hypertension has been unequivocally found to reduce the development of:

- Strokes
- Congestive heart failure
- Probable kidney failure

However, treatment of hypertension has not been shown to reduce heart attacks as well as it has reduced strokes.   There are a number of reasons for this lesser protection against heart attacks, including:

- Heart attacks are caused by more factors than just hypertension such as smoking, high cholesterol and diabetes. Control of hypertension only may not be enough
- The drugs used for treating most hypertension in the past may have aggravated some of the factors responsible for heart attacks, such as cholesterol and blood sugar
- The treatment may not have lowered pressure enough to protect many and may have lowered the pressure too much in some. Either too much or too little could lead to more heart trouble

Clearly, the search is ongoing for better antihypertensive therapy that will protect against all of the cardiovascular consequences of hypertension. The successful treatment of hypertension has undoubtedly played some role in the remarkable decrease in deaths from stroke that has occurred over the last 20 years in the U.S. The lesser, but also very significant, fall in deaths from heart attacks may reflect more the benefits of smoking cessation and lower cholesterol diets.

You do have a great chance to avoid the consequences by successful reduction of your high blood pressure.

#6 Overview of Non-Drug Treatment

Your blood pressure can be reduced more quickly by the use of one or more antihypertensive drugs which may be prescribed by your doctor. But along with or maybe instead of these drugs, you may be able to lower your blood pressure by:

- Losing excess body weight
- Decreasing sodium intake
- Exercising regularly
- Moderating alcohol intake

6. Your physician will decide which drug therapy to use, but the use of various non-drug therapies is largely up to you. An overall non-drug prescription is listed in Table 6.1.

The Treatment That Is Up To You

Whether or not you are asked to take medication to lower your blood pressure, the effective use of non-drug treatments will probably help. For some, non-drug therapy alone may be enough to bring pressure down to a safe level, but likely will be only partially effective. However, you should try non-drug therapy because it:

- Costs nothing
- Causes no side-effects
- May generally benefit your mental and physical health

A word of caution: It takes a large amount of willpower to effectively use non-drug therapies. They require a change in your life-style and sometimes involve breaking habits you have had for many years.

You may not agree that it is worth the effort. It is much easier simply to take one or more pills a day and continue with your present way of life. But all pills may cause some side-effects. Moreover, they may not be effective by themselves in lowering your blood pressure, much less in reducing other risks for early heart disease. Start with a positive, optimistic attitude. Millions of others have helped themselves by using these non-drug treatments, and so can you. Your doctor will help and so will your spouse, family and friends; but, in the end the decision is yours alone. It may not be easy, but it is worth the effort.

Another word of caution: Do not ask too much of yourself. Some people can do it all — stop smoking, lose weight, cut down on sodium, cholesterol, fat, and alcohol, and begin a regular exercise program — but they are exceptional. Although you may want to try a total turnaround, you may be more successful by taking one or or more steps at a time, gaining confidence as you go. Do not give up if you find it tough or slow going. After all, remember how long it took you to become overweight or how long you have been smoking. Do not be surprised if it takes some time to correct these problems. And prepare yourself for occasionally "falling off the wagon." There may be a time when you simply cannot forego those extra calories or that double martini or you just cannot get around to exercising. Do not let that stop you. Accept temporary delays as only that — not as permanent failures.

Additionally, do not let these changes become an obsession that drives you and your family and friends crazy. It is better to stay a bit overweight than to go through life frustrated and constantly bothered by your "weakness."

Begin with confidence. You can accomplish what you attempt. At the same time, be realistic. It may be tough and you may not succeed. By using some of the common-sense ideas that follow, you will look better, feel better and keep your blood pressure under control.

Stop Smoking

Nothing you can do is more important for your health than to stop smoking. It won't lower your blood pressure much, but it will cut your chances of having a heart attack by half or more almost immediately and eventually your chances of lung cancer even more.

Cold turkey is best but the addiction to nicotine is stronger than to cocaine. Therefore, use of gradually decreasing amounts of nicotine (without the other toxins in tobacco smoke) now available in skin patches or chewing gum is a useful way to break the habit. Ask you doctor for help if he or she doesn't ask you to quit.

Meantime, we must do everything possible to keep children from starting to smoke and to becoming addicted to the most harmful addiction ever known - tobacco. One place to start will be to outlaw advertising directed to children, such as Old Joe, the Camel.

TABLE 6.1
OVERALL NON-DRUG PROGRAM

- Reduce excess body weight by caloric restriction. Caution against the use of over-the-counter appetite suppressants — most contain the sympathomimetic phenylpropanolamine which may raise the blood pressure.

- Restrict dietary sodium to 2g per day (or 5g of table salt, sodium chloride), about half the amount in the usual American diet.

- Reduce dietary saturated fat and cholesterol.

- Maintain adequate intake of potassium, calcium and magnesium.

- Limit alcohol intake to less than two ounces and preferably one ounce per day (one ounce of alcohol contained in two usual portions of beer, wine or spirits).

- Perform 20 to 30 minutes of isotonic exercise at least three times a week.

- Use whatever form of relaxation therapy that is acceptable.

- Stop smoking. This will likely not influence the blood pressure but will have a powerfully beneficial effect on overall cardiovascular health.

#7 Weight Reduction

If you are more than 30 pounds overweight, particularly if the extra pounds are in your upper body and abdomen, your obesity probably contributes to your high blood pressure. Although minor degrees of obesity do not pose a health problem by themselves, they often are accompanied by:

- Hypertension
- High cholesterol levels
- A tendency toward diabetes

All of these tendencies are considerable risks to good health.

Everyone can lose some weight, but relatively few can maintain the weight loss. Do not expect too much, too quickly. Frustration soon sets in, and we give up. It is better to try to change your underlying eating habits permanently by carefully thought out behavior modification. To help you start your weight loss program and maintain it, you should:

- Try to lose five or 10 pounds at a time
- Avoid "crash diets"
- Seek help from weight loss organizations
- Become more aware of your present eating habits
- Make eating what it should be — a pleasant way to fulfill biological needs
- Weigh yourself no more than once a week
- Burn more calories than you consume

Losing five or 10 pounds at a time is a goal you can accomplish in one to two months. In so doing, you will feel that you have been successful and can prepare yourself for the next challenge toward reaching your "ideal" weight (Table 7.1).

"Crash diets" may allow you to lose some weight quickly, but they do not teach you improved eating habits that will enable you to keep the weight off. It is better to make sensible changes that will last for the rest of your life—that is how long your weight problem will last.

Remember, you will always have to watch what you eat since you have proven that you will gain weight if your present eating habits are continued. Others may be more fortunate in being able to eat what they want and not gain weight. But for you, a permanent change in eating habits is needed if you are to accomplish permanent weight control.

On the other hand, if you are really obese (more than 50% overweight), you may benefit from a more strenuous program such as a 400-calorie-a-day, modified protein-supplement diet that is very popular today. But if that is what you need, discuss it with your doctor first.

Get all the help you can. Some find Weight Watchers, Take Off Pounds Sensibly (TOPS) and other groups helpful. Others need individual, private assistance from nutritionists, psychologists or others. Ask your doctor's advice.

To become more aware of your present eating habits, it would be beneficial to keep a one-week diary in which you record:

- Everything you eat
- When you eat
- Where you eat
- How much you eat

- How you feel at the time
- All the circumstances surrounding everything that passes your lips

You may be surprised at some of your present compulsive habits, such as your tendency to eat more when you are unhappy or when you are sitting in front of the TV — putting away hundreds of calories without thinking about it, or even enjoying it.

Eating is a biological need which should be enjoyed. To better fulfill this need, keep it a pleasant experience and maintain control of your body weight you should:

- Eat three meals a day, of reasonable pro-
  portions
- Take no second helpings
- Have your plate prepared in the kitchen and
  have no plates of extras placed on the table
- Think about your food, eat it slowly and
  enjoy it — preferably with friends and family
- Quit eating high-calorie snacks between
  meals

However, do not forego little nibbles at appropriate times. At a birthday party, feel free to take a small piece of cake, but leave a little on the plate to show yourself how tough you are.

When the urge is too great, have proper ammunition ready: Carrots, cauliflower or almost any kind of fresh vegetable will keep your mind and mouth busy until the urge passes. Your usual household food stores should not include:

- Candy
- Rich desserts
- Soft drinks

Weigh yourself no more than once a week and do not expect too much. It takes an average deficit of 500 calories a day to lose one pound a week, or a deficiency of 1,000 calories a day to lose two pounds a week (Table 7.2). If you can keep it up, think of what you can do in six months.

While taking in fewer calories, burn more of the ones you take in. This can be accomplished by a regular exercise program, but remember, it takes a lot of exercise to burn a moderate number of calories.

In order for a 150 pound person to burn 400 calories it is necessary to perform one hour of:

- Bicycling 12 miles
- Jogging four miles
- Walking four miles
- Tennis (singles)
- Swimming 40 yards per minute

For every 15 pounds under 150 pounds, subtract 10%; for every 15 pounds over, add 10%.

Regular exercise may do more than help you lose weight. But it may be easier for you, and just as effective in losing weight, if you burn some additional calories while performing your ordinary daily activities. Simple changes will help, such as:

- Parking your car a mile from work and walking the distance
- Walking up and down stairs more often
- Knowing where the extra calories are and substituting lower-calorie foods and drinks
- Cutting away the fat from meat
- Eating more fish and chicken (without the skin)

- Eating more fresh vegetables and salads (with low-cal dressing)
- Substituting fresh fruit for dessert

Use a diet cookbook or other guides. Some are free, such as the pamphlets provided through the American Heart Association. The Association also sells one of the best diet books available for about $18.95.

TABLE 7.1
HOW TO FIGURE YOUR "IDEAL" WEIGHT

Tables are available, but a simple method is to use this formula:

Men — 106 pounds plus six pounds for every inch in height over five feet

Women — 100 pounds plus five pounds for every inch in height over five feet

TABLE 7.2
EXAMPLE OF REASONABLE WEIGHT-LOSS PROGRAM

INTAKE	OUTPUT	RESULTS
t situation 250 calories	2000 calories	250 excess calories per day, or a total of 1750 excess calories per week, will produce 1/2 pound of weight gain per week
program 500 calories	2250 calories	750 calories fewer than output per day, or a total of 5250 calories fewer than output per week, will produce 1-1/2 pounds of weight loss per week

#8 Moderate Sodium Restriction

A reduction in average daily sodium intake by half will lead to a five point (millimeter mercury or mm Hg) or greater fall in blood pressure for about half of all hypertensives. People seem to differ in how sensitive their blood pressure is to either adding or subtracting sodium intake, about half being "sodium sensitive," the other half "sodium insensitive."

Try to reduce sodium intake for four to six weeks and see if your blood pressure is lowered. If so, keep it up; if not, you could go back to your previously high sodium diet. However, in the process you may have lost some of your taste for sodium since it is an acquired taste. Since there is certainly no danger from a modest reduction in sodium intake, it is better to stay on the half-usual amount with hope that it will eventually be helpful. Moreover, others in the family may benefit by the possible effect of the lower sodium intake in preventing the development of hypertension.

Practical Aspects

Sodium content is expressed in milligrams (mg). One flat teaspoonful of sodium chloride (table salt) weighs about 4000 mg, or 4 grams. Of the sodium chloride, a little more than one third is sodium: thus the flat teaspoon of table salt has restrict. Recognize that sodium is present in many forms besides sodium chloride: monosodium glutamate (MSG) is a widely used preservative, baking soda is sodium bicarbonate and sodium carbonate is present in many antacids.

We have already seen that consuming an excessive amount of sodium may possibly be responsible for hypertension. Cutting down sodium intake may, by itself, reduce your blood pressure. Beyond that, a high-sodium intake may decrease the effectiveness of whatever drugs you may have to take.

Your doctor probably does not want you to go on a very low-sodium diet, although such a diet may be needed if you have had heart failure or problems related to excess fluid. A moderate cutback is desirable, to a little less than one half of what you have probably been taking in. That degree of sodium restriction should be possible without much trouble, if you will:

- Quit adding sodium chloride at the table or in cooking
- Cut out obviously salty foods such as pickles, sauerkraut, salted peanuts and country ham
- Watch for sodium that may not be so obvious. Most cheeses are high in sodium, and virtually every food that has been processed (cooked, canned, prepacked) has had sodium added to it (Table 8.1)

Unfortunately, the labels on processed foods must only designate "salt" and not how much has been added. Without knowing the amount, you may be fooled: One 8-ounce can of stewed tomatoes has over 800 mg of sodium, another only 70 mg (Table 8.2).

In summary:

- Eat more fresh foods
- Stay away from obvious salt
- Watch out for hidden sodium, as is found in most canned, frozen and prepackaged foods

Help in cutting down on the hidden sodium in many processed foods will come from new labeling laws in 1993 which will require that the sodium content of all foods be clearly stated on the label. That way you can avoid some of the "salt mines" on the grocery shelf. With a lot of caution and a little concentration, you can easily cut your sodium intake by half.

TABLE 8.1
SODIUM CONTENT OF SOME TYPICAL PROCESSED FOODS

FOOD	SODIUM (mg)
Catsup, 1 tablespoon	156
Tomato juice, 8 ounces	640
Chicken noodle soup, 1 cup	979
Meatloaf TV dinner	1221
McDonald's Big Mac	1510

TABLE 8.2
EXAMPLES OF LOW-SODIUM SUBSTITUTES FOR SOME HIGH-SODIUM FOODS

FOOD	HIGH-SODIUM VERSION	LOW-SODIUM SUBSTITUTE
Green beans, 1 cup	Canned (925 mg)	Fresh (5 mg)
Condiment, 1 teaspoon	Soy sauce (1320 mg)	Lemon juice (0)
Juice, 1 cup	Tomato (640 mg)	Orange (2 mg)
Meat, 3 ounces	Beef frankfurter (425 mg)	Fresh ground beef (57 mg)

#9 Extra Potassium, Calcium and Magnesium

The evidence in favor of increasing the amounts of potassium, calcium and magnesium is not as strong as that in favor of weight reduction and moderate sodium restriction. However, a little more of these minerals should not hurt — and may help.

Potassium

Much of the benefit ascribed to a reduced sodium intake may be the consequence of the increased potassium intake that automatically follows substitution of natural foods (low in sodium, high in potassium) for processed foods (most with sodium added and potassium removed).

We developed our body physiology during thousands of years while our ancestors consumed a diet much lower in sodium and higher in potassium than the "unnatural" high sodium-low potassium diet we now consume (Table 9.1). Therefore it is likely that many of our current cardiovascular problems could result from an inability to handle these marked changes. There seems little to lose and a great deal to possibly gain by going back to a more "natural" diet. Reduce high sodium foods and substitute more natural, high potassium alternatives (Table 9.2).

Calcium

Your diet should contain some low-fat dairy products each day to keep your daily calcium intake around 1000 mg. There is little reason to take more, even if you have thin bones (osteoporosis).

Magnesium

Unless you suffer from chronic alcoholism, diarrheal disorders or some kidney diseases which cause you to waste magnesium, it is likely that you have as much of this mineral as you need and there is no reason for additional supplements.

The other "trace" minerals such as iron, zinc, cobalt, etc. are not involved in the usual types of hypertension. Unless you are on a unique diet, no supplements are needed.

TABLE 9.1 ESTIMATED DIET OF LATE PALEOLITHIC MAN vs. THAT OF CONTEMPORARY AMERICANS

	Late Paleolithic Diet (Assuming 35% Meat)	Current American Diet
Total dietary energy (%)		
Protein	33	12
Carbohydrate	46	46
Fat	21	42
Polyunsaturate: saturate fat ratio	1.41	0.44
Sodium (mg)	690	3400
Potassium (mg)	11000	2400
K/Na ratio	16:1	0.7:1
Calcium (mg)	1500-2000	740

(From Eaton SB, Konner M, Shostak M: Am J Med 84:739, 1988.)

TABLE 9.2
LOW-SODIUM FOODS

Fruits

Apples	Dates (dried)*	Peaches*
Apricots*	Grapefruit*	Pears
Bananas*	Grapes	Pineapple
Cantaloupe*	Honeydew melon*	Plums
Cherries	Oranges*	Watermelon*

Vegetables

Artichokes*	Carrots*	Escarole	Peppers
Asparagus	Cauliflower	Green beans	Potatoes*
Beets	Celery	Lettuce	Spinach
Broccoli*	Corn	Lima beans	Squash
Brussel sprouts*	Cucumber	Mushrooms	Tomatoes*
Cabbage	Eggplant	Peas	Wax beans

Breads and Cereals

Barley	Matzos	Rice
Farina	Noodles	Shredded wheat
Grits	Oatmeal	Tapioca
Low-salt bread, rolls	Puffed rice	Unsalted crackers
Macaroni	Puffed wheat	Unsalted popcorn

Meat, Fish, Poultry (delete pickled, canned and processed forms)

Beef	Veal	Halibut*
Chicken*	Bass	Lobster
Duck	Bluefish	Scallops
Lamb	Cod	Shrimp
Pork	Crab	Sole*
Turkey*	Flounder*	Trout

Seasonings and Flavorings (delete table salt, garlic salt, onion salt, etc.)

Allspice	Cumin	Lime	Pepper
Almond	Curry	Mace	Peppermint
Basil	Dill	Marjoram	Rosemary
Bay leaf	Fennel	Mint	Saffron
Chili powder	Garlic	Onion	Sage
Chives	Ginger	Oregano	Tarragon
Cinnamon	Horseradish	Paprika	Thyme
Cloves	Lemon	Parsley	Vanilla
Coconut			Vinegar

*Also high in potassium.

#10 Fiber and Fats, Alcohol and Caffeine

Fat

Since a high cholesterol level is commonly found in people with high blood pressure, you need to:

- Know that your cholesterol level is normal
- Follow a "prudent" diet to keep your cholesterol at a normal level

A reasonable diet is made up of only 30% fat, considerably below the average 42% in the current American diet. Substitute monounsaturated oils (olive oil is probably the best) for the saturated fats in red meat. Watch out for the few saturated vegetable oils (coconut and palm, in particular) that may be contained in non-dairy cream and added to hundreds of cookies, cakes and fast-foods.

Beyond the benefits of a proper lower-fat diet relative to your cholesterol level, a few studies have shown a fall in blood pressure with lower fat diets.

There are also a few studies showing a fall in blood pressure with extra omega-3-fatty acids obtained from cold water fish. Claims have been made that "omega-3s" protect against heart attacks, presumably because they increase the formation of some hormones (prostaglandins) which help keep blood vessels open and the blood from clotting.

A little aspirin each day (one children's tablet with 80 mg, or one-fourth of what is in a regular aspirin tablet) will likely do all that a large amount of omega-3s can accomplish and the aspirin does not have any calories. Take a children's aspirin tablet every other day unless you are allergic to aspirin.

Fiber

Extra soluble fiber as provided by oat bran will likely lower your cholesterol somewhat.

In a few studies, extra fiber has also been shown to lower blood pressure but it is unknown why this occurs.

Moderation of Alcohol

Besides adding calories, alcohol consumption may raise your blood pressure. One ounce of alcohol per day will probably not raise the blood pressure, but will provide protection against coronary disease and mortality. This can be in the form of either:

- Two beers
- Two glasses of wine
- Two mixed drinks

This has been demonstrated in many epidemiological surveys wherein those who drink one to two ounces of ethanol per day have fewer heart attacks than those who do not drink ethanol.

However, in large population surveys, daily consumption of more than two ounces of alcohol per day is associated with higher blood pressure and more than three ounces per day is often associated with significant hypertension.

#11 Exercise

Regular exercise will help you:

- Lose weight
- Feel better
- Possibly lower your blood pressure

But you should do the correct type of exercise: isotonic, aerobic, dynamic or moving exercise. The other kind, isometric or static exercise, does little other than increase the size of your muscles and may cause your blood pressure to go up considerably while you are doing the isometrics (Figure 11.1). During isotonic exercise (walking, jogging, swimming, etc.) your systolic pressure will go up, but your diastolic pressure will not increase. Actually, it should go down. During isometric exercise, both go up.

To obtain the full "conditioning" effects, you need to do 20 to 30 minutes of strenuous exercise three times a week. The full benefit can be obtained from a level of exercise that increases your pulse to about 70% of maximum. For a 50 year old man that is between 140-160 beats per minute. Before starting such a program, consult your doctor because he may advise you to take it slow until your blood pressure is under reasonable control.

Sexual activity is a form of exercise which need not be curtained by hypertension. Problems may arise, however, that make it difficult for you to enjoy sex. These will be covered in Section #25, Impotence and Other Symptoms.

THE EFFECTS OF ISOMETRIC EXERCISE IN A HYPERTENSIVE PERSON

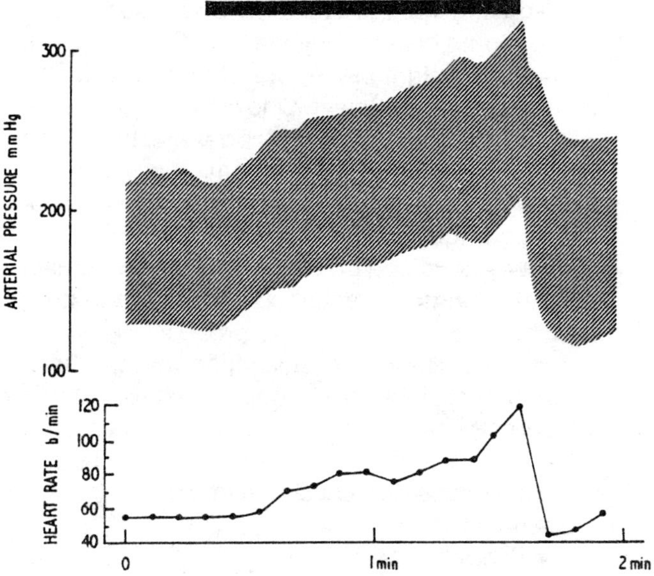

FIGURE 11.1 — The effects of isometric (tension) excerise for one minute in a hypertensive person.

#12 Relaxation

You may want to try a form of relaxation treatment. Some believe they are effective in helping to lower blood pressure, but others have found them to be of little benefit. One of the problems, as with weight reduction, is that many who start such programs do not stick with them. If one is available and you want to try it, your doctor will probably encourage you. But check to see if it is working to lower your blood pressure, and do not neglect the other forms of prescribed non-drug and drug treatment.

Almost all forms of relaxation therapy have been said to lower the blood pressure. These include:

- Progressive muscle relaxation
- Yoga
- Biofeedback
- Transcendental meditation
- The Chinese breathing exercise Qi Gong
- Hypnosis

A few controlled studies have shown a sustained effect beyond the duration of the relaxation procedure. If you are willing to continue the practice of a relaxation therapy, it may help lower your blood pressure.

12.

NOTES

#13 General Guidelines

If your doctor has decided that you need medication to lower your blood pressure, it is likely the non-drug therapies alone are not enough. However, you should still practice as many of the non-drug therapies as possible since they will have additional benefits.

Do not be upset if you need medication. With today's antihypertensive drugs, you can have your blood pressure lowered to a safe level at moderate cost and few side-effects.

To help continue taking your drugs, you should:

- Keep taking your pills even if you feel well
- Maintain your blood pressure below 140/90
- Anticipate the possibility of side effects
- Understand your doctor's directions about:
    - Types of medication (heed labels)
    - Times of day to administer them
    - The precautions about side effects, etc.
- Take your medication as directed
- Not give up if you miss a dose or two
- Not worry about becoming dependent on a drug
- Not take other medications without telling your doctor
- Not change your medications on the basis of home blood pressure readings

Your therapy will almost certainly be life-long. Hypertension rarely is cured unless aggravating factors, such as obesity or consumption of excessive amounts of alcohol, are eliminated. Keep taking your pills even if you feel perfectly well.

Check your pressure every few months even after you have achieved good control. Do not be concerned if it fluctuates somewhat; a change of as much as 20 mm Hg may reflect nothing more than temporary stress or natural variation.

You should anticipate the possibility of occasional, temporary side effects. Any therapy that lowers your pressure may cause you to feel tired and weak temporarily. All therapies may produce some side-effects, as described later. If you are not feeling well, do not stop the therapy and do not skip your next appointment. Call your doctor and discuss the situation with him. Changes in your therapy can almost always be made to overcome any bothersome side effects.

Be sure you understand your doctor's directions about the types of medication and times of the day to take them.

Do not forget to take your medication as directed. If you take one pill a day, take it immediately upon awakening or when you brush your teeth. If you take three or four pills a day, take them before or after meals. Get into the habit of taking you pills routinely at the same time so you do not forget. Many who take multiple doses of one or more pills a day put a day's supply into a pillbox and carry it with them at all times so they will never be caught short.

Do not give up if you happen to miss a dose or two, but do not take all the doses you have missed at one time to make up the loss. Get back on the prescribed schedule.

Do not take other medications without telling your doctor. You may interfere with the control of your hypertension or bring on side effects.

If you and your physician have agreed that you should take your blood pressure at home, follow the directions in the Appendix. Do not change medications on the basis of home readings without checking with your physician.

#14 An Overview of Drug Treatment

There are three major classes of drugs used to treat most hypertension (see Table 14.1):

- Diuretics
- Sympathetic nerve blockers
- Dilators

More are being developed, but if you and your physician work together your blood pressure can almost certainly be controlled with what is now available.

Diuretics

You may be started on a diuretic that causes a temporary increase in urine flow, removing some excess sodium and water from your body (Figure 14.1).

Sympathetic Nerve Blockers

Sympathetic nerve blockers act in different sites to slow the activity of the sympathetic nerves, which are part of the autonomic nervous system. This autonomic nervous system keeps the:

- Heart beating
- Lungs inflating
- Bowels moving

Since part of their function is to increase the force of the heartbeat and to tighten the blood vessels, it is easy to see how partially blocking the activity of these nerves will also lower the blood pressure.

14.

Dilators

The third class of drugs acts directly on the blood vessel walls to open them further, thus allowing the pressure of the blood within the vessels to fall. Others of this same class are used intravenously to treat very severe hypertension.

In addition to the direct dilators, two newer classes of drugs act by dilating the blood vessels. These drugs are:

- Angiotensin converting enzyme (ACE) inhibitors
- Calcium entry blockers

These two classes are growing rapidly in popularity and are replacing some of the older sympathetic nerve blockers.

In the next few chapters, each of these different types of drugs will be described, with emphasis on some side effects that may be encountered.

TABLE 14.1
TYPES OF DRUGS USED TO TREAT HYPERTENSION

(available in U.S. as of April, 1992)

GENERIC NAME	TRADE NAME
Diuretics	(see Table 15.1)
Thiazides	
Loop diuretics	
Potassium sparers plus diuretic	
Sympathetic blockers	
Peripherally acting	
Bethanidine	Tenathan
Guanadrel	Hylorel
Guanethidine	Ismelin
Rauwolfia derivatives	Raudixin
	Rauwiloid
	Reserpine
Centrally acting	
Clonidine	Catapres
Guanabenz	Wytensin
Guanfacine	Tenex
Beta-blockers	
Acebutolol	Sectral
Atenolol	Tenormin
Betaxolol	Kerlone
Carteolol	Cartrol
Metoprolol	Lopressor
Nadolol	Corgard
Penbutolol	Levatol
Pindolol	Visken
Propranolol	Inderal
Timolol	Blocadren

Continued ⇨

TABLE 14.1 – (Continued)
TYPES OF DRUGS USED TO TREAT HYPERTENSION
(available in U.S. as of April, 1992)

GENERIC NAME	TRADE NAME
Alpha-blockers	
Doxazosin	Cardura
Prazosin	Minipress
Terazosin	Hytrin
Alpha- and Beta-blocker	
Labetalol	Normodyne, Trandate
Direct Dilators	
Hydralazine	Apresoline
Minoxidil	Loniten
Converting enzyme inhibitor	
Benazepril	Lotensin
Captopril	Capoten
Enalapril	Vasotec
Fosinopril	Monopril
Lisinopril	Prinivil, Zestril
Quinapril	Accupril
Ramipril	Altace
Calcium entry blocker	
Diltiazem	Cardizem
Felodipine	Plendil
Isradipine	Dynacirc
Nicardipine	Cardene
Nifedipine	Procardia
Verapamil	Calan, Isoptin

The Effects of Antihypertensive Medications on the Blood Pressure

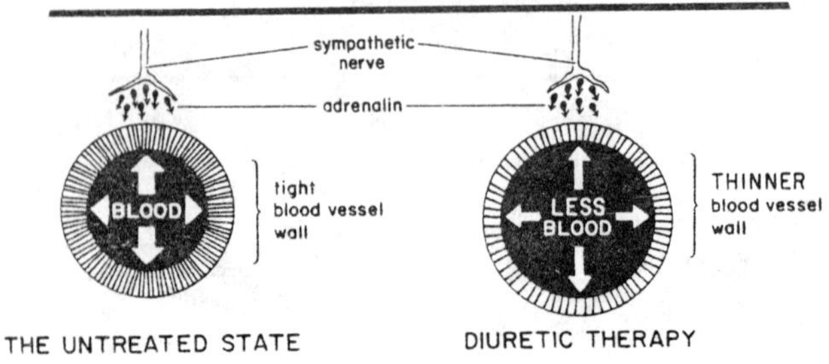

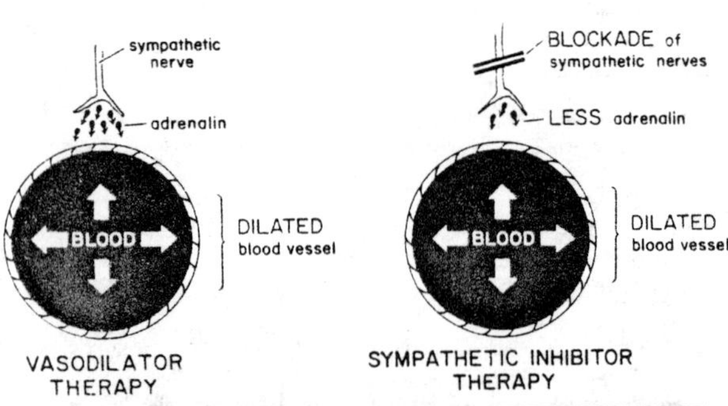

FIGURE 14.1 — A stylized representation of the effects of the three major types of antihypertensive medications on the blood pressure. The untreated state (upper left) involves an overfilled, tight circulation. With diuretic therapy (upper right), excess sodium and fluid are excreted, reducing the amount of circulation and thinning the blood vessel walls. With vasodilator therapy (lower left), the vessel walls are directly dilated. With sympathetic blocking drugs (lower right), the vessels dilate because they are relieved of some of the constriction previously caused by activity of the sympathetic nerves.

NOTES

1.	The Normal Blood Pressure	**What Is Hypertension**
2.	What do the Numbers Mean?	
3.	Why Does the Blood Pressure Go Up?	
4.	What are the Consequences of High Blood Pressure?	
5.	Can Hypertension be Prevented?	
6.	Overview of Non-Drug Treatment	**Treating Hypertension Without Drugs**
7.	Weight Reduction	
8.	Moderate Sodium Restriction	
9.	Extra Potassium, Calcium and Magnesium	
10.	Fiber and Fats, Alcohol and Caffeine	
11.	Exercise	
12.	Relaxation	
13.	General Guidelines	**Treating Hypertension With Drugs**
14.	An Overview of Drug Treatment	

Treating Hypertension With Drugs (continued)	Diuretics and Potassium Sparers	15.
	Sympathetic Blockers: Peripheral and Central	16.
	Sympathetic Blockers: Alpha and Beta	17.
	Calcium Entry Blockers	18.
	Angiotensin Converting Enzyme (ACE) Inhibitors	19.
	Other Antihypertensive Drugs	20.
Treating Special People and Problems	Diabetics	21.
	Heart Disease	22.
	Cerebral Disease	23.
	Kidney Disease	24.
	Impotence and Other Symptoms	25.
	Elderly	26.
	Children	27.
	Taking your own Blood Pressure	28.

#15 Diuretics and Potassium Sparers

THIAZIDE DIURETICS

A large number of diuretics, all of which increase the excretion of sodium and water, are available (Table 15.1).   Additionally, there are three drugs (potassium sparing agents) which are used with diuretics to hold potassium in the body which would otherwise be excreted with a diuretic.

The moderately long-acting diuretic hydrochlorothiazide (HCTZ) is the most popular drug in the United States for therapy of hypertension.

To lower the blood pressure, diuretics must initially increase excretion of sodium and water, which shrinks blood volume. Continued diuretic use leads to a fall in peripheral vascular resistance which is the major reason for the continued antihypertensive effect.

Most patients will achieve a 10 mm Hg fall in blood pressure with daily therapy. Those with more "volume dependent" hypertension tend to respond particularly well. These include many black and elderly hypertensives.

Side Effects

A number of side effects accompany the use of diuretics. Despite the long list of potential problems, diuretics have proven to be effective and generally safe when used in the lowest dose needed and with proper surveillance of biochemical changes.

Some side effects are allergic or idiosyncratic, such as skin rash. More common are a variety of biochemical changes, which in large part reflect an exaggeration of the expected, desired effect of the drugs.

Low Blood Potassium (Hypokalemia)

Increased excretion of potassium is usual with diuretic therapy, and this may lower the amount of potassium in the blood to below normal, referred to as hypokalemia.

Hypokalemia rarely causes symptoms, although muscular weakness and leg cramps may be noted. However, an increase in heart rhythm irregularity may occur.

Diuretic-induced hypokalemia can be minimized by these steps:

- Use the smallest dose of diuretic possible
- Reduce dietary sodium intake to 2 g per day
- Increase dietary potassium intake
- Combine potassium-sparers with the diuretic

Elevation in Blood Cholesterol (Hypercholesterolemia)

A moderate increase in total serum cholesterol may develop and persist for years unless countered by reduction of saturated fat in the diet.

Elevation in Blood Sugar (Glucose Intolerance)

Fasting and postprandial blood sugars may rise but diabetes rarely develops.

Elevation in Blood Uric Acid (Hyperuricemia)

The diuretic decreases the excretion of one of the waste products, uric acid, leading to its elevation in the blood or hyperuricemia. Usually diuretic-induced hyperuricemia need not be treated even if plasma levels rise above 10 mg/dl. However, susceptible people may develop gout which usually shows up as a very painful arthritis, often in the big toe.

Other biochemical problems may rarely develop, including a rise in blood calcium (hypercalcemia), which actually could be helpful in people with kidney stones caused by increased excretion of calcium in the urine. Less calcium is excreted in a manner similar to uric acid, usually raising blood calcium levels slightly.

A significant fall in the amount of sodium in the blood is rarely noted, usually in elderly patients who are given too much diuretic.

Despite these multiple potential problems, most people have no problems when taking a daily diuretic.

LOOP DIURETICS

With more severe hypertension, particularly with associated kidney damage, a more potent diuretic may be needed.

The two agents now available, furosemide (Lasix) and bumetanide (Bumex), are short acting with their effect lasting three to six hours. They must be given two to three times a day to maintain the slight shrinkage of body volume needed to keep the blood pressure down.

POTASSIUM-SPARING AGENTS

Three potassium-sparing agents are now available. Spironolactone blocks the action of the hormone, aldosterone, that causes potassium to be excreted. The other two, triamterene and amiloride, simply block potassium excretion into the urine.

These three potassium-sparers are almost always used in combination with the thiazide diuretic, hydrochlorothiazide (HCTZ). Their common names are:

- Spironolactone + HCTZ = Aldactazide
- Triamterene + HCTZ = Dyazide or Maxzide
- Amiloride + HCTZ = Moduretic

TABLE 15.1
DIURETICS

Thiazides
  Bendroflumethiazide (Naturetin)
  Benzthiazide (Aquatag, Exna)
  Chlorothiazide (Diuril)
  Cyclothiazide (Anhydron)
  Hydrochlorothiazide (Esidrix, HydroDiuril, Oretic)
  Hydroflumethiazide (Saluron)
  Methyclothiazide (Enduron)
  Polythiazide (Renese)
  Trichlormethiazide (Metahydrin, Naqua)

Related sulfonamide compounds
  Chlorthalidone (Hygroton)
  Indapamide (Lozol)
  Metolazone (Zaroxolyn, Diulo)

Loop diuretics
  Bumetanide (Bumex)
  Furosemide (Lasix)

Potassium-sparing agents
  Amiloride (Midamor)
  Spironolactone (Aldactone)
  Triamterene (Dyrenium)

NOTES

#16 Sympathetic Blockers:
Peripheral and Central

The second significant class of drugs inhibits the activity of the sympathetic nervous system which has two major components:

- Alpha-receptors
- Beta-receptors

As shown in Table 16.1, the primary sites of action vary from the brain to the peripheral nerves. Some block the alpha-receptors and others block the beta-receptors.

The peripheral-acting agents include reserpine, which acts in the central nervous system (CNS) as well as upon peripheral nerves. These drugs are among the longest-used antihypertensives, but have lost much popularity as other agents have become available.

CENTRALLY-ACTING AGENTS

These drugs, including Aldomet and Catapres, have been among the more popular drugs used to treat hypertension. They dampen centers within the brain which control the level of activity of the sympathetic nervous system. As a result, the heart's pumping action is decreased slightly but the main effect is to dilate the blood vessels. Although the four currently available members of this group differ, they share a common mechanism of action and side effects.

Side Effects

Because they act in the brain, sedation and dryness of the mouth are frequently noted side effects. Beyond these, there are few side effects.
This class of drugs seems particularly attractive for those people who:

- Can tolerate or escape their sedative action
- Would likely not do well with beta-blockers or diuretics

These include:

- Elderly patients
- Diabetics
- Hypercholesterolemics
- Those with asthma
- Those having peripheral vascular disease

TABLE 16.1 CHARACTERISTICS OF SYMPATHETIC BLOCKER

Drug	Trade Name	Side Effects
Peripheral:		
Reserpine	Serpasil	Sedation, nasal congestion, depression
Guanethidine	Ismelin	Orthostatic hypotension, diarrhea
Guanadrel	Hylorel	Orthostatic hypotension
Central:		
Methyldopa	Aldomet	Sedation, liver dysfunction, fever, "auto-immune" disorders
Clonidine	Catapres	Sedation, dry mouth, "withdrawal hypertension"
Guanabenz	Wytensin	Sedation, dry mouth, dizziness
Guanfacine	Tenex	Sedation, dry mouth, dizziness
Alpha-blocker:		
Doxazosin	Cardura	Postural hypotension (mainly with first dose), lassitude
Prazosin	Minipress	Postural hypotension (mainly with first dose), lassitude
Terazosin	Hytrin	Postural hypotension (mainly with first dose), lassitude
Beta-blockers:		
Acebutolol	Sectral	Serious: bronchospasm, congestive heart failure,
Atenolol	Tenormin	masking of insulin-induced
Betaxolol	Kerlone	hypoglycemia, depression

Continued ⇓

TABLE 16.1 CHARACTERISTICS OF SYMPATHETIC BLOCKER (Continued)

Drug	Trade Name	Side Effects
Beta-Blockers *(cont.)* Carteolol Metoprolol Nadolol Penbutolol Pindolol Propranolol Timolol	Cartrol Lopressor Corgard Levatol Visken Inderal Blocadren	Less Serious: poor peripheral circulation, insomnia, slow heart rate, fatigue, decreased exercise tolerance, hypertriglyceridemia, decrease HDL-cholesterol
Combined Alpha- and Beta-blocker Labetalol	Normodyne Trandate	Postural hypotension, beta-blocking side effects

#17 Sympathetic Blockers:
Alpha and Beta

The multiple actions of the sympathetic nerves that automatically control various body functions are expressed through receptors (or keys) on the cells that are activated (or turned) when they are stimulated. There are two main types of sympathetic nervous receptors:

- Alpha
- Beta

Different mechanisms are involved in activating these two receptors; one slowing down, the other speeding up a given body function.

Blood pressure can be reduced by blocking either the alpha receptors or the beta receptors, in quite different ways.

ALPHA-BLOCKERS

These drugs, including Cardura, Minipress and Hytrin, block actions of the sympathetic nerves that involve the alpha-component. In doing so, they lower blood pressure by causing blood vessels to dilate.

The dilation of blood vessels that occurs with the first dose of an alpha-blocker may be so significant as to cause the pressure to fall excessively. To avoid a "first-dose low-pressure," the alpha-blocker should be taken at a time when you do not need to stand up soon thereafter, preferably on going to bed.

Beyond this uncommon problem, some continue to notice dizziness with an alpha-blocker.

BETA-BLOCKERS

Members of this group of drugs have become the second most popular after diuretics. They lower blood pressure mainly by slowing the heart rate and force of heart contraction, thereby decreasing the pump action that is responsible for the pressure of fluid within the blood vessels (see Section #1). Since these drugs "relax" the heart muscle, they are also widely used to treat coronary disease (angina) and heart rhythm irregularities. The are also frequently given after a heart attack.

There are a number of beta-blockers. All lower the blood pressure to an approximate equal degree and share most side effects. The more common side effects seen with beta-blockers are:
- Easy fatigue and decreased ability to exercise, related to a decreased output of blood from the heart
- Bad dreams and fitful sleep
- A rise in blood triglyceride levels
- Precipitation of asthma and other allergies

ALPHA- AND BETA-BLOCKER

One drug, labetalol (Normodyne or Trandate) combines both alpha- and beta-blocking actions, thereby reducing the blood pressure by both slowing heart action and dilating blood vessels (but mainly by the latter). It is used mainly to treat more severe degrees of hypertension, but can be given to patients with milder disease as well.

The main side effect is too low a blood pressure on standing (postural hypotension). Other problems seen with beta-blockers may also be seen with this drug.

#18 Calcium Entry Blockers

This group of drugs lowers blood pressure by dilating blood vessels. They do so by blocking the entry of calcium from the blood into the muscular cells that make up the blood vessel wall. In order for these cells to contract and thereby reduce the diameter of the blood vessel and raise the pressure within the circulation, calcium must enter to act as the signal for contraction. Calcium entry blockers, as the name implies, block the entry of calcium into the muscular cells of the blood vessels, preventing their contraction and thereby keeping the vessels open or dilated and lowering the blood pressure. These drugs have a relatively specific effect on the blood vessels, with little action on the muscular cells of the heart, intestines, uterus or skeletal muscles.

Since they dilate the blood vessels supplying the heart muscle, they are also widely used in the treatment of coronary artery disease (angina). Also, as they dilate the blood vessels in the kidneys, they may cause a slight increase in urine flow.

Types of Calcium Entry Blockers

There are three main types of these drugs, each blocking calcium entry in a somewhat different way, but each lowering the blood pressure about the same. They differ not only chemically but also in their side effects. These three types are:

- Verapamil — the first of these discovered and now in use for over 20 years

- Diltiazem
- A family of dihydropyridines, including nifed-
  ipine, nicardipine and a number of others

Side Effects

The most frequent side effect of these three types of calcium entry blockers are:

- Verapamil
  - Constipation
  - Dizziness upon standing (postural hypo-
    tension)
  - Headache
- Diltiazem
  - Side effects similar to verapamil
  - Less constipation
- Dihydropyridines
  - Flushing
  - Headache
  - Swelling around the ankles

Special Benefits

For most patients, these drugs are effective and free of side effects. Since they do not cause the biochemical side effects of diuretics (low potassium, high cholesterol) or of beta-blockers (high triglycerides), they are becoming more widely used as first line treatment for all degrees of hypertension. They seem to be particularly effective in elderly patients.

Because these drugs also have a mild diuretic action, they usually work well without a diuretic. They can be combined with other antihypertensive agents if needed.

#19 Angiotensin Converting Enzyme (ACE) Inhibitors

This is the most recently introduced family of antihypertensive drugs and, along with the calcium entry blockers, are fast becoming popular for treatment of all degrees of hypertension. They can be given alone as the first drug or combined with a diuretic which will usually lead to a further reduction of the blood pressure.

These drugs also lower blood pressure by dilating the blood vessels but differently than the calcium entry blockers. The ACE inhibitors block the action of one of the circulating hormones, renin-angiotensin, which comes from the kidneys and which directly constricts the blood vessels throughout the body. The activation of renin-angiotensin requires the intervention of an enzyme called the angiotensin converting enzyme (ACE). The ACE inhibitors prevent the ACE from working, thereby blocking the action of renin-angiotensin and allowing blood vessels to dilate so that blood pressure falls.

Types of ACE Inhibitors

As of Mid 1992, seven of these drugs are available:

- Benazepril (Lotensin)
- Captopril (Capoten)
- Enalapril (Vasotec)
- Fosinopril (Monopril)
- Lisinopril (Prinivil or Zestril)
- Quinapril (Accupril)
- Ramipril (Altace)

They are approximately equal in blood pressure lowering effectiveness and side effects but they do have some subtle differences that could be important. For most hypertensive patients, any of the seven (or of the additional ones which are likely to soon be available) will lower the blood pressure, again with few side effects.

Side Effects

The manufacturers of ACE inhibitors have demonstrated that they cause less interference with the quality of life than do centrally-acting agents, e.g. Aldomet, or beta-blockers, e.g. Inderal. But, they may cause a:

- Dry, hacking cough
- Measles-like skin rash
- Loss of taste sensitivity

Some dizziness upon standing (postural hypotension) may be seen, particularly after the first dose, because they quickly and effectively lower blood pressure. Less common is kidney damage or a fall in white blood cells in the blood.

Special Benefits

ACE inhibitors may have some special benefits in protecting the heart muscle after a heart attack and the kidneys in patients with diabetes. They are also being widely used to treat congestive heart failure since they reduce the work load imposed on the weakened heart muscle.

#20 Other Antihypertensive Drugs

A number of drugs are currently being tested and some may be approved by the Food and Drug Administration (FDA) after they have been shown to be both effective in lowering blood pressure and free from serious side effects in carefully performed clinical trials.

In the meantime, a number of other dilating drugs are available, some for use only in severe life-threatening hypertensive emergencies where they are usually given intravenously. These include:

- Nitroprusside
- Nitroglycerine
- Trimethaphan
- Diazoxide
- Some I.V. forms of oral drugs previously mentioned, e.g. labetalol.

DIRECT DILATORS

There are also two more dilating drugs, hydralazine (Apresoline) and minoxidil (Loniten), which are effective by mouth and are used usually as the third drug when two do not prove adequate to bring the pressure down enough. These agents dilate the blood vessels in a different manner than do ACE inhibitors or calcium entry blockers and are referred to as "direct dilators." When they act, they tend to stimulate both the sympathetic nervous system and renin-angiotensin so they need to be given with diuretics and sympathetic blockers to maintain their effectiveness.

Minoxidil was found to stimulate hair growth all over the body when used internally to lower blood pressure.

Side Effects of Direct Dilators

Most side effects of direct dilators are related to their significant dilation of blood vessels, including:

- Flushing and headache—opening up of blood vessels in the face and head
- Fast heart beat—reflex increase in sympathetic nerve activity in an attempt to bring the pressure up by constricting the blood vessels and stimulating the heart
- Skin rash, painful joints—usually developes only when high doses of Hydralazine (Apresoline) are administered
- Increased growth of body hair—use of Minoxidil (Loniten). If this side effect is undesirable, the drug can be stopped and most of the excess hair rapidly falls out

These drugs may be helpful in treating more severe degrees of hypertension, particularly with associated kidney damage. They are seldom used for milder forms by hypertension.

20.

#21 Diabetics

Hypertension is found about twice as often among people with diabetes. When it is present, hypertension tends to aggravate the kidney and eye damage that frequently develops with long-standing diabetes. Hypertension is particularly common when diabetes develops in older obese women, but it may be a problem in diabetics of any age.

Problems with Antihypertensive Drugs

Although it is important to keep blood pressure under good control, there are numerous special problems with various antihypertensive drugs. These problems call attention to the need for weight reduction and the other non-drug therapies covered in Sections #6 through #12 in order to help both the diabetes and the hypertension. Some examples of problems in diabetics with antihypertensive drugs are:

- Diuretics may raise the blood sugar further
- Beta-blockers may prolong the duration of episodes of low blood sugar (hypoglycemia) that may occur with the use of insulin. Also, the usual warning signals of an impending low blood sugar episode (hunger, fast heart beat, shakiness) may not be noted. Sweating still occurs and can be used as the signal that a low sugar spell is developing
- Both diuretics and beta-blockers may further elevate blood lipid levels which tend to be high in diabetics

- Diabetics may develop dizziness upon standing (postural hypotension) as a result of nerve damage; this can be aggravated by antihypertensives which dilate blood vessels

Despite these possible problems, careful control of hypertension appears to be vital in order to prevent or slow the damage to the eyes and kidneys as well as the narrowing of blood vessels in the heart and extremities that so often occur in long-standing diabetes.

Careful use of any drug may successfully control the hypertension seen in diabetics. However, calcium entry blockers and ACE inhibitors are being used increasingly since they may work well without inducing some of the side effects seen with other drugs.

21.

#22 Heart Disease

The widespread and effective treatment of hypertension is partially responsible for the fall in deaths from various cardiovascular disorders noted over the past 20 years in the U.S. However, heart attacks still remain the leading cause of death.

Coronary Artery Disease

Partial obstruction of the arteries supplying the heart muscle, by cholesterol and fat-containing plaques, may lead to angina—pain arising from an oxygen-deprived heart muscle. Angina usually appears when extra demands are placed on the heart, as during:

- Exercise
- Emotional distress
- Eating

If the obstruction becomes complete, usually by a blood clot forming on top of a fatty plaque, the heart muscle supplied by the blocked artery suffers a heart attack or myocardial infarction.

Clot dissolvers are now available and, if given soon after start of the attack, the artery can be re-opened before the heart muscle dies.

If you have coronary disease and hypertension, treatment will usually include one or more of these:

- Nitrates, e.g. nitroglycerine—dilates the coronary arteries to allow more blood to pass beyond the partial blockage
- Calcium entry blockers—also dilate coronary arteries but in a different manner
- Beta-blockers—decreases the work required by the heart muscle

For many coronary patients, the obstructions can be mechanically opened by a balloon (angioplasty) or by by-pass surgery.

Congestive Heart Failure

After many years of overwork, the heart muscle may not be able to pump hard enough to maintain a normal flow of blood. Blood backs up behind the weakened heart, mainly in the lungs, leading to shortness of breath. Later the fluid builds up in the legs as edema. The process is called congestive heart failure.

The weakened heart can be strengthened by either:

- Decreasing the demand placed upon it by removing excess fluid or dilating the arteries so the heart has to work less. This can be accomplished by administering:
  - Diuretics
  - ACE inhibitors
- Increasing the efficiency of the heart muscle with heart stimulants — primarily digitalis

Enlargement of the Heart

Long before heart failure develops, the heart muscle becomes progressively thicker in order to perform the extra work of pumping blood against a high blood pressure. The enlarged or hypertrophied heart muscle (left ventricle) may give rise to irregular heart rhythm and, if its blood supply is not adequate, angina. Fortunately, successful reduction of the blood pressure is often followed by a decrease in the size of the enlarged heart.

#23 Cerebral Disease

Strokes are the end result of damage to the blood vessels supplying the brain, i.e. cerebrovascular disease.   Hypertension is the major risk factor for the development of cerebrovascular disease or accident (CVA). The number of strokes has been markedly reduced by successful treatment of hypertension.

Types of Stroke

There are three major types of strokes:

- Hemorrhage — the most dramatic event is a hemorrhage due to rupture of a blood vessel. If it affects only a small vessel supplying a non-critical area of the brain, recovery is possible
- Thrombus — if the blood vessel is blocked by a locally formed clot (thrombus), the stroke is only a little less dramatic but its consequences are similar
- Embolus — a third possibility is an embolus, a clot that arises elsewhere, usually within the heart or blood vessels in the neck, and ends up blocking a blood vessel in the brain

In many patients, partial blockage of the arteries in the neck (the carotids) may lead to transient ischemic attacks (TIAs), wherein the blood supply is interrupted only transiently. The area of the brain made ischemic (deficient in blood supply) does not function properly so that the following symptoms may suddenly occur:

- Weakness
- Loss of sensation
- Loss of vision

The process is usually temporary and normal brain function returns. However, TIAs are warning signals for a complete stroke.

Treatment of Hypertension With Cerebral Disease

If you have cerebrovascular disease and hypertension, it is important to control the blood pressure carefully, avoiding both too-high pressures which continue to damage the fragile vessels in the brain as well as too-low pressures which diminish the supply of blood through already narrowed vessels.

Effective treatment can be provided with an antihypertensive medication. Proceed slowly so as not to reduce the blood supply acutely. In the presence of a very high pressure, however, rapid reduction may be needed to protect cerebral vessels from further acute damage.

In addition to antihypertensive medications, daily aspirin therapy has been shown to reduce the development of strokes in patients with TIAs.

#24 Kidney Disease

Hypertension is now the leading cause for chronic kidney failure, referred to as end-stage renal disease (ESRD). In the U.S., over 100,000 people are receiving chronic dialysis therapy for ESRD, removing the waste products by artificial filtering devices which the kidneys are no longer capable of removing. Many patients on kidney dialysis are able to receive a kidney transplant from a donor (living relative or someone who died very recently), thereby restoring adequate kidney function to lead a normal life.

Hypertension as a Cause of Kidney Disease

Long-standing hypertension may damage the small blood vessels throughout the kidneys, causing loss of function in the areas supplied by these vessels. The problem is seen most frequently among black hypertensives. The process is usually recognized first by the presence of protein in the urine, reflecting damage to the kidney tissue. Later, waste products build up in the blood, the serum creatinine level being the easiest to measure.

Kidney Disease as a Cause of Hypertension

Various diseases can damage the kidneys so that they can no longer remove enough of the sodium and water consumed daily, the build-up overfilling the circulation and raising the blood pressure. Numerous diseases can affect the kidneys. In the past, nephritis or Bright's disease was most common. Now, diabetes is second only to hypertension. In addition, injury from various drugs (including pain relievers such as phenacetin) is also a fairly common cause for chronic kidney damage.

Treatment

Kidney disease and hypertension frequently coexist. The successful treatment of hypertension will almost certainly slow the progression of kidney damage. The treatment of hypertension in the presence of mild kidney damage can usually be provided by diuretics which squeeze out more of the excess fluid through the still responsive kidneys.

As kidney damage worsens, more potent antihypertensive agents are needed including minoxidil (Loniten) and stronger diuretics may be used. When the kidneys quit working, dialysis must be started to take over their function.

24.

#25 Impotence and Other Symptoms

Hyperventilation

The psychological burden of knowing that you have hypertension may lead to various problems, including anxiety-induced acute hyperventilation. The inadvertent over-breathing changes in the body chemistry, leading to many of the symptoms ascribed to hypertension. These include:

- Headaches
- Dizziness
- Numbness and tingling in the hands
- Difficulty swallowing with a sensation of a lump in the throat
- Chest discomfort
- Palpitations
- A feeling of shortness of breath.

These symptoms are quite real and may make the unsuspecting patient even more anxious, leading to a viscious cycle: anxiety causes hyperventilation which causes more anxiety. The cycle can be broken if you understand what is happening and if you rebreathe into a paper sack for a minute or so to overcome the chemical changes which triggered the entire process.

Impotence

Impotence (the inability to gain and maintain an erection) may have a psychological basis. Obviously this is a male problem although the female partner is very much affected.

If you are a hypertensive male, impotence may arise for four reasons:

- First, you may be intimidated into impotence simply by being told that you have high blood pressure

- Second, occasional impotence may occur at any age. Once again, it may reflect psychological causes, such as:
  - Too much stress
  - Feelings of inadequacy
  - Too much alcohol
  - The feeling that you are "over the hill"
- Third, some of the antihypertensive drugs can cause impotence. Discuss any pre-medication difficulties with your doctor, and certainly report any problems that develop
- Fourth, a real decrease of blood flow into the penis may result from partial obstruction by atherosclerotic plaques similar to those seen in other blood vessels so that an erection cannot occur. As elsewhere, these plaques develop more in the presence of:
  - Hypertension
  - High blood cholesterol
  - Cigarette smoking
  - Diabetes

A number of therapies are available, including:
- Rings that hold blood within the penis
- Injections of drugs that increase blood flow
- Various surgical procedures

No one need suffer from persistent impotence. If it is psychogenic, it can be overcome. If it is caused by antihypertensive medication, it can almost always be relieved by a change to another which will more gradually reduce the blood pressure and allow blood flow to the penis to be well maintained. If it is from organic interruption to blood flow, various therapies are available. Talk to your physician or contact a urological specialist.

25.

#26 Elderly

People develop more hypertension as they grow older (Figure 26.1). Among those over 65, much of the hypertension is purely systolic, that is only the upper number becomes elevated. Readings such as 190/80 mm Hg may be seen.

The mechanism for what is called "isolated systolic hypertension (ISH) in the elderly" is different than the combined systolic and diastolic hypertension in younger and middle-aged people.

During the aging process, the large arteries, including the major one leading from the heart (the aorta), become increasingly more rigid as their walls become thickened by the presence of atherosclerotic plaques. The rigidity prevents the large arteries from expanding to hold the blood pumped out with each heart beat. Therefore, the systolic pressure rises increasingly placing an additional burden on these already hardened arteries, leading to more ruptures of their walls and obstructions to the flow of blood.

Only recently, scientific proof has become available that lowering isolated systolic pressures in the elderly can reduce the likelihood of various vascular complications. It appears that elderly people may actually gain even more protection from strokes and heart attacks from carefully lowering of high blood pressure than can younger people.

However, slow, gentle and gradual treatment is needed to lower systolic pressures to below 160 mm Hg. Treatment can be provided with the drugs described in previous chapters. Calcium entry blockers are becoming particularly popular. There are, however, some special problems:

- Older people may be prone to dizziness upon standing (postural hypotension) and this can be worsened by some drugs
- Large doses of diuretics may reduce body fluids too much
- Drug dosages may need to be reduced because of reduced kidney function which causes them to stay in the body longer
- Other drugs used to treat other common problems may interfere with the action of antihypertensive agents. The non-steroidal anti-inflammatory drugs (NSAIDs) commonly used to treat arthritis, e.g. Motrin, Ibuprofen, Feldene, etc., are examples

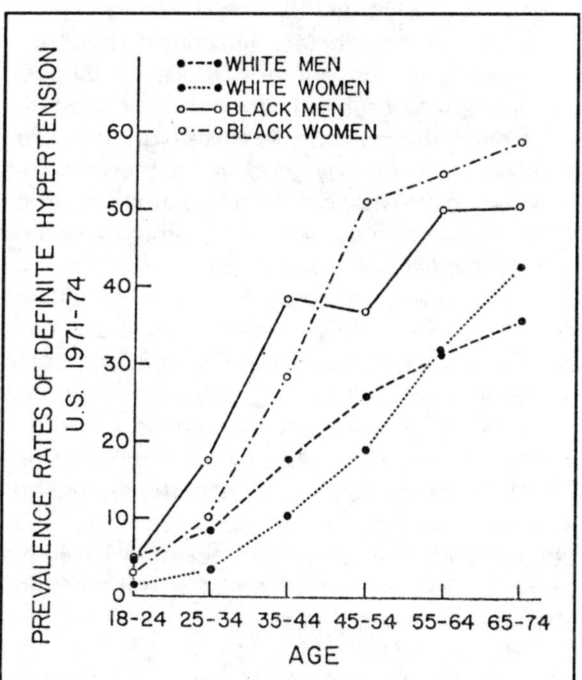

FIGURE 26.1 — The increasing prevalence of hypertension with advancing age in the various groups in the U.S.

26.

#27 Children

A few young children have hypertension which is usually secondary to a congenital defect in the kidneys or to a partial blockage in the main artery leading from the heart (coarctation of the aorta). These problems usually show up as poor growth and development and often require surgery.

In children after puberty, hypertension becomes more common so that as many as one per 100 adolescents aged 14 to 18 will have hypertension. Hypertension usually is the same unknown type (essential or primary) as seen in over 90% of adults with hypertension.

Obesity is a major factor in causing hypertension in children. Weight reduction is most important in managing obese hypertensive children.

Unless the pressure is quite high, non-drug therapies are usually tried since there is little experience with the use of antihypertensive drugs with children and there are concerns about their possible effects on normal growth and development. However, if needed, drugs should be used since serious cardiovascular complications have been seen in children with severe, untreated hypertension.

One problem sometimes noted in young athletes is an elevated systolic blood pressure, with a reading such as 150/75. Most of these readings are related to a temporary rapid, overactive heart action which may be psychogenic and they are probably of no consequence. However, caution should be advised against:

- Heavy isometric exercise (see Section #11)
- The use of anabolic steroids
- Any alcohol consumption

Hopefully, the high systolic pressures will go down on repeated measurements and aerobic exercise can safely be performed.

27.

#28 Taking Your Own Blood Pressure

If your physician suggests that you measure your own blood pressure at home, follow these directions.

Equipment

- Sphygmomanometer — blood pressure gauge (manometer) attached to a balloon that is encased in a rigid cloth cuff. A bulb is attached to fill the balloon with air
- Stethoscope — listening device to amplify sounds

A number of "home" sphygmomanometers and stethoscopes are available, costing from about $25 to $200. The more expensive models do all of the work, inflating and releasing the air from the balloon and recording the pressure by a display on a small screen. The following instructions are for the less expensive, do-it-yourself models with an air (aneroid) gauge and a stethoscope for hearing the sounds. Semi-automatic devices that only need to be inflated manually are now available for around $50 and are much easier to use, with no need for using a stethoscope or reading a gauge. For most, they are preferable.

The pressure gauge on the home device should be checked against a manometer with a mercury column, which is almost certainly accurate. This can be done in your physician's office simply by connecting the two instruments with a Y-tubing to the same pressure source. If you have a large arm, your physician may suggest using a larger cuff with a wider and longer balloon.

Technique

Before trying this yourself, you may have your physician or nurse demonstrate the technique and check the accuracy of your reading. You may find it more practical to have your spouse or some other person take your pressure.

The proper time and place for checking your pressure may vary. For most people, the best time will be soon after rising from a night's sleep. Another time that may be useful is during stressful periods.

If you are taking medications, it will be useful to take your pressure at varying times of the day to see if the drug's effects last all day. Thereafter, take your pressure under the same circumstances to monitor the long-term course of your blood pressure.

Follow these steps to obtain accurate readings:

1. Place the cuff with the deflated balloon around your arm, with its lower edge about one inch above your elbow. If you are right-handed, it will be easier for you to take the pressure in your left arm. Either arm may be measured.

2. If you use a separate, detached stethoscope, place it just below the crease of the elbow and just to the inside of the middle of your forearm, over the main artery. Feel for the pulsation of this artery in the area. If you cannot find it, ask your physician to show you.

28.

3.   Be sure the cuff is snug. If it remains in place
     when you lower your arm, it is tight enough.
     Your arm should rest comfortably on a table or
     arm of a chair.

4.   Be sure the bulb is in a closed, screwed-down
     position so the air does not leak out. Then
     inflate the balloon quickly by squeezing the
     rubber bulb rapidly and tightly.

5.   To be sure you have raised the pressure in the
     balloon above the systolic pressure, feel your
     pulse at the wrist, and note that it disappears
     when the pressure in the balloon is above the
systolic pressure. It is preferable to raise the
     balloon pressure about 20 mm Hg above the
     systolic pressure. No sounds should be heard
     through the stethoscope when you are above
     the systolic pressure.

6.   Begin to deflate the balloon by letting a little air
     out, barely opening the screw at the base of
     the rubber bulb. The pressure should fall no
     more than three to five points (millimeters of
     mercury) per heartbeat.

7.   As the pressure falls, listen for the first thump-
     ing sounds through the stethoscope. When
     the first sounds appear, read the gauge. That
     is the systolic pressure.

8.   Continue to let the air out of the balloon. The
     thumping sounds will change somewhat and
     may become quite faint. As long as you can
     hear them, you are still above the diastolic
     pressure. The sounds should be distinct until
     they suddenly disappear.

Read the pressure on the gauge when the sounds disappear. That is the diastolic pressure.

9. You should take a second reading after a two minute wait. If the two pressures vary more than 10 mm Hg, relax a few minutes and try a third time. Some real fluctuations in your pressure may occur, and a variation of 10 mm Hg between readings is not unusual. If the third reading is fairly close to one of the first two, take the average of the two closer readings.

10. Finally, do not become anxious and start checking your pressure excessively. But do check your pressure if you:

    • Feel dizzy or faint upon standing
    • Have a bad headache
    • Want to see what the effect of an emotional outburst or a period of exercise has on your pressure

Do not panic if your pressure changes considerably under such conditions, but let your physician know what you have discovered.

Used properly, home blood pressure readings can be extremely helpful in controlling hypertension. Once you have learned to take accurate readings, check the blood pressures of the members of your family and your friends. If you find pressure elevated above 140/90, advise that person to see his or her physician.